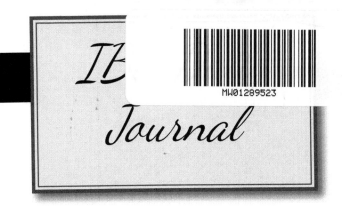

SUZANNE PERAZZINI

Creator of *Strands of My Life*

www.strandsofmylife.com
lowfodmapcoach@gmail.com

© 2015

Copyright

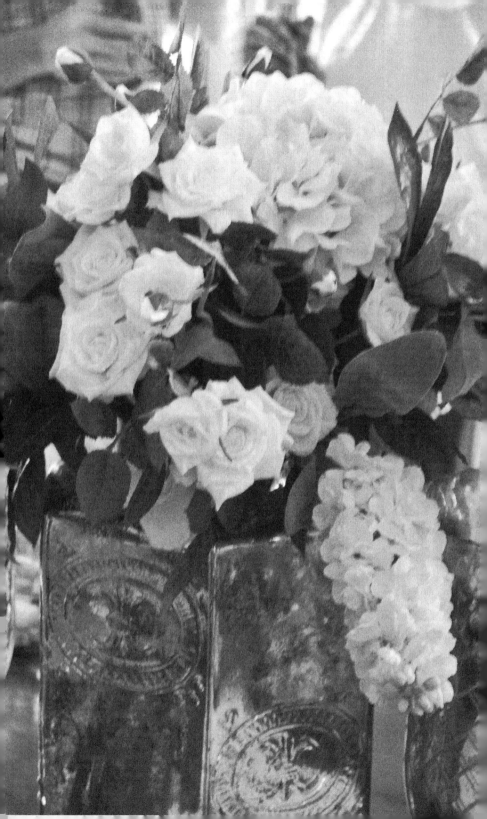

Contents

4   HOW TO USE THIS JOURNAL

6   BREAKFAST

8   SNACKS

9   LUNCH

10   DINNER

11   MEDICATION

12   SUPPLEMENTS

13   WATER

14   BOWEL MOVEMENTS

15   BRISTOL STOOL CHART

16   THE JOURNAL

The best way to work out what is happening with your digestive system is to record all the relevant information. Record every single thing that goes into your mouth including medication and supplements. Record your bowel movements, what sort they are and when they happen.

On top of that, record how much sleep you get, how much exercise you do and when you use relaxation techniques. These are essential parts of a balanced lifestyle which supports your IBS.

As time passes, this will be an excellent record to look back on to see what progress you have made. But most of all, it will be a way for you to start seeing patterns and work out what is causing your symptoms.

Assuming you are on a strict low Fodmap diet, this will be a fairly easy process because your symptoms will be minimal. However, there could still be some foods that upset you for reasons which are not Fodmap related. Or maybe you will see that too much of something or too many low Fodmap foods together are causing symptoms.

We are all individuals where Fodmaps are concerned, and it is rare for a person to have issues with all the Fodmap groups so you will be able to create your perfect personalized diet over time, especially once you have undertaken the reintroduction stage of the diet.

Make sure you eat five small meals a day spaced between three and five hours apart with your last meal at least three hours before bedtime. Never overeat, do not to graze throughout the day and do not to fast. All of these situations will cause your IBS symptoms to reappear or worsen. Follow the diet strictly and you will be amazed at how your IBS symptoms will disappear. Record, learn and adjust. Good luck.

"Courage doesn't always roar.
Sometimes courage is the little voice at the end of the day that says I'll try again tomorrow."
ary Anne Radmacher

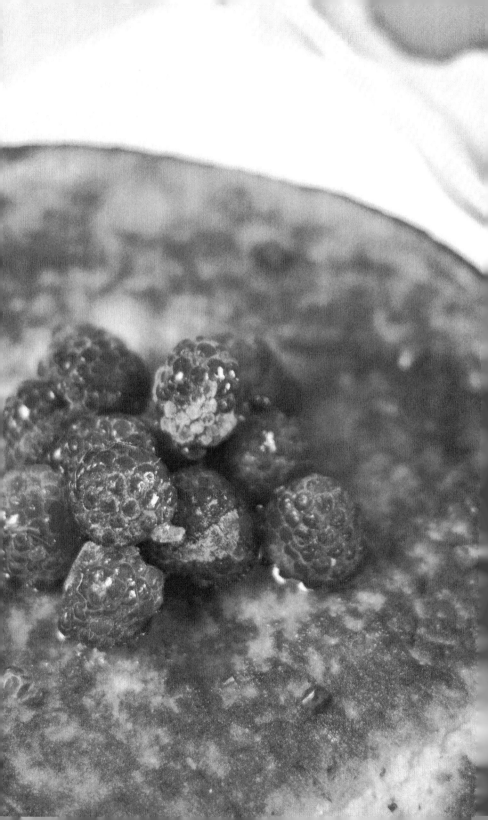

Breakfast

You should consume your breakfast as soon as you get up or perhaps after a shower. Breakfast, as the word says, breaks the fast. And it's important with IBS to do that as soon as possible. Our digestive systems hate to feel starved and react with symptoms. The food arriving into the digestive system will also activate the urge to have a bowel movement, and it is great to get that out of the way before the day fully starts.

WHAT SHALL I EAT?

A good choice is a wheat/barley/rye-free cereal like oatmeal [1/4 cup when raw], cornflakes [3/4 cup], rice flakes [3/4 cup] etc., a low Fodmap fruit and lactose-free milk. Weak tea or coffee is optional. If you need more protein that the milk will provide, have an egg prepared how you prefer. If you are on the constipated side of IBS, I suggest oats and a kiwifruit, which has a mild laxative effect.

RECORD

Take note in your diary pages, what you eat, how much and when you eat. Note how you feel after eating.

TIP: Check the ingredients of any cereal you choose and make sure you recognize all the ingredients as low Fodmap.

Snacks

You need to have two snacks a day in between your main meals and you need to keep all meals small since our digestive systems don't like large amounts of food arriving at the same time. Make sure you have the first snack 3-5 hours after your breakfast and keep that same spacing for your meals throughout the day, making sure that your dinner is at least three hours before bedtime. If you get up late, still have your breakfast straightaway and perhaps skip the morning snack. But distribute any important food from the snack into your other meals so you are not eating less.

WHAT SHALL I EAT?
Homemade baking would be suitable. But some good alternatives are a few of the following - low Fodmap fruit (2-3 pieces a day), low Fodmap vegetable sticks, cottage cheese, hard cheese, peanut butter, tahini, canned fish, gluten-free crackers, lactose-free yogurt.

RECORD
Take note in your diary pages, what you eat, how much and when you eat it. Also note how you feel after eating the meal.

TIP: The best combination is to have a protein, a carbohydrate and a fruit or vegetable sticks so that you don't get hungry.

Lunch

Lunch is your third meal of the day and should be 3-5 hours after your morning snack. Make sure you stop work or whatever you are doing and take a complete break so you can focus on eating your food. Any kind of stress or tension will affect how the food is received

WHAT SHALL I EAT?

Eating leftover dinner is the easiest way to take care of lunch whether you are eating at home or at work. Most work places have microwaves so you can heat it up. If there are no leftovers or 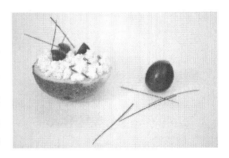 if they are not suitable, a gluten-free sandwich with fresh sliced meat and low Fodmap salad vegetables would be a good alternative.

RECORD

Take note in your diary pages, what you eat, how much and when you eat it. Also note how you feel after eating the meal.

TIP: Before you eat your dinner, put aside your lunch so that it doesn't get eaten.

Dinner

Eat your dinner 3-5 hours after your afternoon snack and at least three hours before bed. When planning your dinner, make sure it has protein, carbohydrate and vegetables. Carbohydrate gives you instant energy which doesn't last long while the energy from protein takes a little longer to kick in but lasts longer. Combining the two at all five meals is ideal for keeping away hunger, which is your enemy. Eat in a calm situation and don't gulp air while you eat.

WHAT SHALL I EAT?

This depends on your preferences. However, as above, make sure you balance your meal well with all food groups while staying low Fodmap. This is the largest meal of the day in many cultures, but you have to cut back on what you would usually eat because now your food is being distributed between five meals instead of the traditional three.

RECORD

Take note in your diary pages, what you eat, how much and when you eat it. Also note how you feel after eating the meal.

> TIP: Vary your proteins between red meat, chicken, fish, tofu etc. throughout the week.

Medication

Those on the low Fodmap diet sometimes forget that everything they swallow affects their gut, and that includes medication.

Some medication are lifesaving and can't be stopped. But that medication may contain high Fodmap inactive ingredients so do have a chat with your doctor and ask about all the ingredients in the medicine you are taking. It could be possible to make a change if necessary.

Many with IBS are on anti-depressants because they haven't been absorbing tryptophan, which plays a part in regulating a person's moods. This situation will gradually change as you start to actually absorb the nutrients in your food. And so those medicines can be reduced under the careful supervision of your doctor – because many of them are habit-forming and the withdrawal from them has to be done with care.

Many medicines have common side effects that affect the gut and so it's almost impossible to know if it is food or pills that are causing symptoms. This is a very tricky situation and has to be handled with care.

TIP: Having a doctor who fully understands your personal situation and understands the concepts of the low Fodmap diet will go a long way to helping you resolve these problems together. If your doctor is uncooperative and doesn't listen to your concerns, change doctor.

Supplements

Many people with IBS are taking a whole raft of supplements in an attempt to get better. And that is very understandable. But most of them will be unnecessary once you are eating a diet which is healthy for you because you will finally be absorbing all the nutrients in your food.

Some supplements contain high Fodmaps, and it takes some work to find the very best supplements which won't hurt your gut. Regard every single thing that goes down into your gut with suspicion and do your research into them all. Google 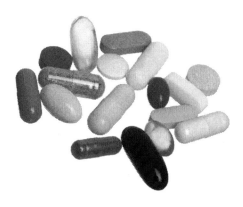 the ingredients and side effects of these things, become informed about what you are consuming and talk to your doctor or chemist about any doubts you have.

RECORD

TIP: Look for an ingredient ending in "ol" - it could be one of the Fodmap groups, a Polyol.

Water

Water is needed by every sytem in our body and makes up 60% of our body weight. Even mild dehydration will make us listless and tired.

HOW MUCH WATER DO YOU NEED?
That depends on a variety of things:
- How much exercise you do? An athlete will require more fluid than someone who only walks each day.

- Location is important. Hot temperatures cause loss of fluids through perspiration. Even heated interiors dry out your skin. Higher altitudes also cause a greater loss of hydration through increased respiration and urination.

- Some illnesses like a bladder infection or a tummy bug with diarrhea cause dehydration.

On average a man requires 3 litres and a woman needs 2.2 litres of fluid a day.

RECORD
Make note of how many glasses you drink in a day and when you drank them.

TIP: Drink a glass of water with each of your 5 meals and a glass in between each meal.

Bowel Movements

During the elimination and reintroduction stages of the diet, it is important to monitor your bowel movements carefully and make adjustments to your diet according to your stools that day. On the next page you will see the Bristol Stool Chart. This is the generally accepted measure of a person's stools. Our aim is to have

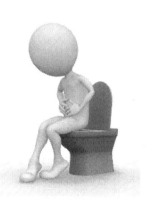

a number 3 or 4 stool on a regular basis. This means that we are neither constipated nor have diarrhea. The average person has one to three bowel movements a day. But some people have one every two days or four movements a day. You have to find what is right for you.

Create a routine that your body comes to recognize but the very best time to go is staright after breakfast before starting your day. If you need a second visit, make it just before bedtime so that you can have a good settled night's sleep. A third time, if necessary, could be straight after lunch.

TIP: Don't ignore an urge to visit the toilet especially if you are constipated. That can make the condition worse.

Bristol Stool Chart

Type 1		Separate hard lumps, like nuts - hard to pass
Type 2		Sausage-shaped but lumpy
Type 3		Like a sausage but with cracks on the surface
Type 4		Like a sausage or snake, smooth and soft
Type 5		Soft blobs with clear-cut edges
Type 6		Fluffy pieces with ragged edges, a mushy stool
Type 7		Watery, no solid pieces. Entirely liquid

Personal Challenge

Tell someone close to you that you love them

Date: 8 / 5 / 17

Sleep   7.00 hours   From 11:30 to 6:30

Quality of sleep _____

Exercise   _____ hours   From _____ to _____

Type _____

Relaxation   _____ minutes   From _____ to _____

Type _____

Meal	Time	Notes/Symptoms
Breakfast gluten free bread Ham mozzarella lactose free milk	7:00 Am	Ø Symptoms
Morning Snack gluten free granola	10:00 Am	Ø Symptoms
Lunch mashed potatoes chicken	12:00 Am	Abdominal pain Some bloating
Afternoon Snack gluten free cookies	4:00 pm	Ø Symptoms
Dinner		
Medication		
Supplements		
Total glasses of water /X//		
Bowel Movements Morning afternoon	6:00 Am 6:00 pm.	

ají
oregano
verduritas
Tomates

oregano?
verduritas?

Date: 8 / 5 / 17

Sleep   8 ½ hours   From 11:30 to 8:00

Quality of sleep _____ Good. _____

Exercise _____ hours   From _____ to _____

Type _____

Relaxation _____ minutes   From _____ to _____

Type _____

Meal	Time	Notes/Symptoms
Breakfast gluten free bread mozzarella Ham lactose free milk	9:30	Ø
Morning Snack —		
Lunch cheese with crackers	2:00 pm	Ø
Afternoon Snack		
Dinner crab salad with fries Lager · Soy Ice cream later	6:00 pm	Ø
Medication Peppermint capsules Probiotics omeprazole.		
Supplements		
Total glasses of water		
Bowel Movements 2		

Gratitude Affirmation

*I gratefully accept all the good
that manifests in my life.*

Date: 8 / 6 / 12

Sleep   8 : 20 hours   From 10:40 to 7:00

               Quality of sleep _____ good _____

Exercise   _____ hours   From _____ to _____

               Type _____

Relaxation   _____ minutes   From _____ to _____

               Type _____

Meal	Time	Notes/Symptoms
Breakfast wheat bread mozzarella. Bread with peanut Butter	7.30 & 10:00 Am	Today I had. abdominal pain & 3 B.M. maybe from Yesterday Stay ice cream???
Morning Snack		
Lunch arroz + pollo	2:00	Ø Symptoms
Afternoon Snack granola		Ø Symptom
Dinner papa + huevo	6:30	Ø Symptom
Medication		
Supplements		
Total glasses of water		
Bowel Movements I I I		

Bananas are rich in potassium which can be good for keeping your blood pressure healthy.

Date: 8 / 9 / 17

Sleep _____ hours   From _____ to _____

Quality of sleep _____

Exercise 1 : 40 hours   From _____ to _____

Type _Running_ / Cardio _____

Relaxation _____ minutes   From _____ to _____

Type _____

Meal	Time	Notes/Symptoms
Breakfast no Gluten Free Bread MOZZARELLA Turkey Ham	7:00A —	Ø Symptoms
Morning Snack Luna Bar macadamia + white chocolate		Ø
Lunch chicken + Rice	12:30	Ø
Afternoon Snack —		
Dinner mash potatoes + Fried egg + lager	9:00 p —	Ø
Medication omeprazole	7:00 A —	
Supplements		
Total glasses of water		
Bowel Movements 2		

Personal Challenge

Smile at 3 strangers today

Date: 8 /10 / 17

Sleep _7:45_ hours From _10:45_ to _6:30_

Quality of sleep _Good but Had a Headache._

Exercise _____ hours From _____ to _____

Type _____

Relaxation _____ minutes From _____ to _____

Type _____

Meal	Time	Notes/Symptoms
Breakfast Bread Gluten Free Jam Cheese	7:00A —	∅
Morning Snack		
Lunch Rice & Salmon	12:00	∅ Bloating & pain afterwards
Afternoon Snack		
Dinner Potatoes & cheese	7:00	∅
Medication		
Supplements		
Total glasses of water		
Bowel Movements 3		

Quote

"We have to live life with a sense of
urgency so not a minute is wasted."
Les Brown

Date: 8 / 12 / 17

Sleep _____ hours   From _____ to _____

Quality of sleep _____

Exercise _____ hours   From _____ to _____

Type _____

Relaxation _____ minutes   From _____ to _____

Type_____

Meal	Time	Notes/Symptoms
Breakfast gluten free bread ham cheese (cheddar)	8:00A —	∅
Morning Snack chips (corn)		∅
Lunch Tacos with chicken & pico de gallo (Tomato, onion, cilantro)	2:00	afterwards had abdominal pain
Afternoon Snack		
Dinner gluten free cheese pizza		∅
Medication Bentyl x 1		
Supplements		
Total glasses of water		
Bowel Movements 2		

Gratitude Affirmation

My gratitude is sincere and constant.

Date: 8 / 13 / 17

Sleep _____7_____ hours From __11:00__ to __6:00__

Quality of sleep _____

Exercise _____ hours From _____ to _____

Type _____

Relaxation _____ minutes From _____ to _____

Type _____

Meal	Time	Notes/Symptoms
Breakfast Bread * Ham + cheese		Ø
Morning Snack		
Lunch noodle rice & chicken		Ø
Afternoon Snack		
Dinner mash potatoes & Eggs		Ø
Medication		
Supplements		
Total glasses of water		
Bowel Movements 3		

Bowel movements were painful &
hot mixture. I'm Thinking it was
The onion from the Pico de Gallo.

Health Tip

A red pepper has nine times more vitamin C than a green one.

Date: 8 / 15 / 17

Sleep   7:20 hours   From 11:00 to 6 20

Quality of sleep   Good

Exercise   30 minutes hours   From _____ to _____

Type   Running

Relaxation   _____ minutes   From _____ to _____

Type _____

Meal	Time	Notes/Symptoms
Breakfast Gluten Free bread Ham cheese		∅
Morning Snack Granola		bloating
Lunch chicken & Rice		3 bloating from granola
Afternoon Snack		
Dinner mashed potatoes + egg		∅
Medication		
Supplements		
Total glasses of water		
Bowel Movements 3		

Granola has been an issue. 2 different
ones have caused bloating

Personal Challenge

Don't complain for an entire day

Date: ___/___/___

Sleep   _____ hours   From _____ to _____

                     Quality of sleep _____

Exercise   _____ hours   From _____ to _____

               Type _____

Relaxation   _____ minutes   From _____ to _____

               Type_____

Meal	Time	Notes/Symptoms
Breakfast		
Morning Snack		
Lunch		
Afternoon Snack		
Dinner		
Medication		
Supplements		
Total glasses of water		
Bowel Movements		

Date: ___/___/___

Sleep _____ hours   From _____ to _____

Quality of sleep _____

Exercise _____ hours   From _____ to _____

Type _____

Relaxation _____ minutes   From _____ to _____

Type _____

Meal	Time	Notes/Symptoms
Breakfast		
Morning Snack		
Lunch		
Afternoon Snack		
Dinner		
Medication		
Supplements		
Total glasses of water		
Bowel Movements		

Sleep   _____ hours   From _____ to _____

                         Quality of sleep _____

Exercise   _____ hours   From _____ to _____

                Type _____

Relaxation   _____ minutes   From _____ to _____

                Type_____

Meal	Time	Notes/Symptoms
Breakfast		
Morning Snack		
Lunch		
Afternoon Snack		
Dinner		
Medication		
Supplements		
Total glasses of water		
Bowel Movements		

Health Tip

Stretching when you wake up boosts circulation and digestion.

Date: ___/___/___

Sleep   _____ hours   From _____ to _____

                  Quality of sleep _____

Exercise   _____ hours   From _____ to _____

           Type _____

Relaxation   _____ minutes   From _____ to _____

           Type_____

Meal	Time	Notes/Symptoms
Breakfast		
Morning Snack		
Lunch		
Afternoon Snack		
Dinner		
Medication		
Supplements		
Total glasses of water		
Bowel Movements		

Personal Challenge

Carve your name on a tree in your garden.

Date: ___/___/___

Sleep   _____ hours   From _____ to _____

Quality of sleep _____

Exercise   _____ hours   From _____ to _____

Type _____

Relaxation   _____ minutes   From _____ to _____

Type _____

Meal	Time	Notes/Symptoms
Breakfast		
Morning Snack		
Lunch		
Afternoon Snack		
Dinner		
Medication		
Supplements		
Total glasses of water		
Bowel Movements		

"Live as big as you can, with what you've got."
Jill Shalvis

Date: ___/___/___

Sleep _____ hours   From _____ to _____

Quality of sleep _____

Exercise _____ hours   From _____ to _____

Type _____

Relaxation _____ minutes   From _____ to _____

Type _____

Meal	Time	Notes/Symptoms
Breakfast		
Morning Snack		
Lunch		
Afternoon Snack		
Dinner		
Medication		
Supplements		
Total glasses of water		
Bowel Movements		

Gratitude Affirmation

With every breath I take, I am bringing more and more gratitude into my life.

Date: ___/___/___

Sleep _____ hours   From _____ to _____

Quality of sleep _____

Exercise _____ hours   From _____ to _____

Type _____

Relaxation _____ minutes   From _____ to _____

Type_____

Meal	Time	Notes/Symptoms
Breakfast		
Morning Snack		
Lunch		
Afternoon Snack		
Dinner		
Medication		
Supplements		
Total glasses of water		
Bowel Movements		

Date: ___/___/___

Sleep _____ hours   From _____ to _____

Quality of sleep _____

Exercise _____ hours   From _____ to _____

Type _____

Relaxation _____ minutes   From _____ to _____

Type _____

Meal	Time	Notes/Symptoms
Breakfast		
Morning Snack		
Lunch		
Afternoon Snack		
Dinner		
Medication		
Supplements		
Total glasses of water		
Bowel Movements		

Personal Challenge

Sing in the shower at the top of your voice

Date: ___/___/___

Sleep _____ hours From _____ to _____

Quality of sleep _____

Exercise _____ hours From _____ to _____

Type _____

Relaxation _____ minutes From _____ to _____

Type_____

Meal	Time	Notes/Symptoms
Breakfast		
Morning Snack		
Lunch		
Afternoon Snack		
Dinner		
Medication		
Supplements		
Total glasses of water		
Bowel Movements		

Quote

"Be determined enough to live for your dreams."
Lailah Gifty Akita

Date: ___/___/___

Sleep _____ hours From _____ to _____

Quality of sleep _____

Exercise _____ hours From _____ to _____

Type _____

Relaxation _____ minutes From _____ to _____

Type_____

Meal	Time	Notes/Symptoms
Breakfast		
Morning Snack		
Lunch		
Afternoon Snack		
Dinner		
Medication		
Supplements		
Total glasses of water		
Bowel Movements		

Gratitude Affirmation

I am grateful for all my material possessions

Date: ___/___/___

Sleep _____ hours   From _____ to _____

Quality of sleep _____

Exercise _____ hours   From _____ to _____

Type _____

Relaxation _____ minutes   From _____ to _____

Type _____

Meal	Time	Notes/Symptoms
Breakfast		
Morning Snack		
Lunch		
Afternoon Snack		
Dinner		
Medication		
Supplements		
Total glasses of water		
Bowel Movements		

Health Tip

Never skip breakfast. An IBS gut hates fasting through the day.

Date: ___/___/___

Sleep   _____ hours   From _____ to _____

               Quality of sleep _____

Exercise   _____ hours   From _____ to _____

           Type _____

Relaxation   _____ minutes   From _____ to _____

           Type_____

Meal	Time	Notes/Symptoms
Breakfast		
Morning Snack		
Lunch		
Afternoon Snack		
Dinner		
Medication		
Supplements		
Total glasses of water		
Bowel Movements		

Personal Challenge

Do something you used to love doing when you were a small child

Date: ___/___/___

Sleep _____ hours   From _____ to _____

Quality of sleep _____

Exercise _____ hours   From _____ to _____

Type _____

Relaxation _____ minutes   From _____ to _____

Type _____

Meal	Time	Notes/Symptoms
Breakfast		
Morning Snack		
Lunch		
Afternoon Snack		
Dinner		
Medication		
Supplements		
Total glasses of water		
Bowel Movements		

Quote

"Live with passion. Live with enthusiasm. Live your best life."
Lailah Gifty Akita

Date: ___/___/___

Sleep   _____ hours   From _____ to _____

Quality of sleep _____

Exercise   _____ hours   From _____ to _____

Type _____

Relaxation   _____ minutes   From _____ to _____

Type _____

Meal	Time	Notes/Symptoms
Breakfast		
Morning Snack		
Lunch		
Afternoon Snack		
Dinner		
Medication		
Supplements		
Total glasses of water		
Bowel Movements		

Gratitude Affirmation

I find it easy to maintain an attitude of gratitude even in difficult situations

Date: ___/___/___

Sleep   _____ hours   From _____ to _____

Quality of sleep _____

Exercise   _____ hours   From _____ to _____

Type _____

Relaxation   _____ minutes   From _____ to _____

Type_____

Meal	Time	Notes/Symptoms
Breakfast		
Morning Snack		
Lunch		
Afternoon Snack		
Dinner		
Medication		
Supplements		
Total glasses of water		
Bowel Movements		

Date: ___/___/___

Sleep   _____ hours   From _____ to _____

         Quality of sleep _____

Exercise   _____ hours   From _____ to _____

      Type _____

Relaxation   _____ minutes   From _____ to _____

      Type_____

Meal	Time	Notes/Symptoms
Breakfast		
Morning Snack		
Lunch		
Afternoon Snack		
Dinner		
Medication		
Supplements		
Total glasses of water		
Bowel Movements		

Personal Challenge

Do something that scares you

Date: ___/___/___

Sleep _____ hours   From _____ to _____

Quality of sleep _____

Exercise _____ hours   From _____ to _____

Type _____

Relaxation _____ minutes   From _____ to _____

Type _____

Meal	Time	Notes/Symptoms
Breakfast		
Morning Snack		
Lunch		
Afternoon Snack		
Dinner		
Medication		
Supplements		
Total glasses of water		
Bowel Movements		

"A heart can no more be forced to love than a stomach can be forced to digest food by persuasion."
Alfred Nobel

Date: ___/___/___

Sleep _____ hours   From _____ to _____

Quality of sleep _____

Exercise _____ hours   From _____ to _____

Type _____

Relaxation _____ minutes   From _____ to _____

Type_____

Meal	Time	Notes/Symptoms
Breakfast		
Morning Snack		
Lunch		
Afternoon Snack		
Dinner		
Medication		
Supplements		
Total glasses of water		
Bowel Movements		

Gratitude Affirmation

I am so grateful for every person and every thing in my life.

Date: ___/___/___

Sleep   _____ hours   From _____ to _____

Quality of sleep _____

Exercise   _____ hours   From _____ to _____

Type _____

Relaxation   _____ minutes   From _____ to _____

Type _____

Meal	Time	Notes/Symptoms
Breakfast		
Morning Snack		
Lunch		
Afternoon Snack		
Dinner		
Medication		
Supplements		
Total glasses of water		
Bowel Movements		

Health Tip
20 minutes of sunshine covers your daily vitamin D needs or eat plenty of fatty fish, eggs, beef liver and cheese

Date: ___ / ___ / ___

Sleep _____ hours   From _____ to _____

Quality of sleep _____

Exercise _____ hours   From _____ to _____

Type _____

Relaxation _____ minutes   From _____ to _____

Type _____

Meal	Time	Notes/Symptoms
Breakfast		
Morning Snack		
Lunch		
Afternoon Snack		
Dinner		
Medication		
Supplements		
Total glasses of water		
Bowel Movements		

Personal Challenge

Show someone how much you love them.

Date: ___/___/___

Sleep _____ hours   From _____ to _____

Quality of sleep _____

Exercise _____ hours   From _____ to _____

Type _____

Relaxation _____ minutes   From _____ to _____

Type_____

Meal	Time	Notes/Symptoms
Breakfast		
Morning Snack		
Lunch		
Afternoon Snack		
Dinner		
Medication		
Supplements		
Total glasses of water		
Bowel Movements		

Quote

"We must live life and treasure every moment on Earth."
Lailah Gifty Akita

Date: ___/___/___

Sleep _____ hours   From _____ to _____

Quality of sleep _____

Exercise _____ hours   From _____ to _____

Type _____

Relaxation _____ minutes   From _____ to _____

Type_____

Meal	Time	Notes/Symptoms
Breakfast		
Morning Snack		
Lunch		
Afternoon Snack		
Dinner		
Medication		
Supplements		
Total glasses of water		
Bowel Movements		

My life is singular, unique and wondrous. For this I am profoundly thankful.

Date: ___ / ___ / ___

Sleep _____ hours   From _____ to _____

Quality of sleep _____

Exercise _____ hours   From _____ to _____

Type _____

Relaxation _____ minutes   From _____ to _____

Type _____

Meal	Time	Notes/Symptoms
Breakfast		
Morning Snack		
Lunch		
Afternoon Snack		
Dinner		
Medication		
Supplements		
Total glasses of water		
Bowel Movements		

Health Tip

Rev up your metabolism by alternating your speed and intensity during aerobic workouts.

Date: ___/___/___

Sleep _____ hours   From _____ to _____

Quality of sleep _____

Exercise _____ hours   From _____ to _____

Type _____

Relaxation _____ minutes   From _____ to _____

Type_____

Meal	Time	Notes/Symptoms
Breakfast		
Morning Snack		
Lunch		
Afternoon Snack		
Dinner		
Medication		
Supplements		
Total glasses of water		
Bowel Movements		

Personal Challenge

Brush your teeth with your non-dominant hand. This is excellent for exercising the brain.

Date: ___/___/___

Sleep   _____ hours   From _____ to _____

Quality of sleep _____

Exercise   _____ hours   From _____ to _____

Type _____

Relaxation   _____ minutes   From _____ to _____

Type _____

Meal	Time	Notes/Symptoms
Breakfast		
Morning Snack		
Lunch		
Afternoon Snack		
Dinner		
Medication		
Supplements		
Total glasses of water		
Bowel Movements		

Date: ___/___/___

Sleep _____ hours   From _____ to _____

Quality of sleep _____

Exercise _____ hours   From _____ to _____

Type _____

Relaxation _____ minutes   From _____ to _____

Type_____

Meal	Time	Notes/Symptoms
Breakfast		
Morning Snack		
Lunch		
Afternoon Snack		
Dinner		
Medication		
Supplements		
Total glasses of water		
Bowel Movements		

Gratitude Affirmation

My thoughts are focused on positivity and thankfulness

Date: ___/___/___

Sleep _____ hours   From _____ to _____

Quality of sleep _____

Exercise _____ hours   From _____ to _____

Type _____

Relaxation _____ minutes   From _____ to _____

Type_____

Meal	Time	Notes/Symptoms
Breakfast		
Morning Snack		
Lunch		
Afternoon Snack		
Dinner		
Medication		
Supplements		
Total glasses of water		
Bowel Movements		

Health Tip
Laughter boosts the immune system and helps the body shake off allergic reactions. It heals bodies as well as broken hearts.

Date: ___/___/___

Sleep   _____ hours   From _____ to _____

              Quality of sleep _____

Exercise   _____ hours   From _____ to _____

           Type _____

Relaxation   _____ minutes   From _____ to _____

           Type_____

Meal	Time	Notes/Symptoms
Breakfast		
Morning Snack		
Lunch		
Afternoon Snack		
Dinner		
Medication		
Supplements		
Total glasses of water		
Bowel Movements		

Personal Challenge

Hold the door open for two people today

Date: ___/___/___

Sleep _____ hours   From _____ to _____

Quality of sleep _____

Exercise _____ hours   From _____ to _____

Type _____

Relaxation _____ minutes   From _____ to _____

Type_____

Meal	Time	Notes/Symptoms
Breakfast		
Morning Snack		
Lunch		
Afternoon Snack		
Dinner		
Medication		
Supplements		
Total glasses of water		
Bowel Movements		

"Worry is the stomach's worst poison."
Alfred Nobel

Date: ___/___/___

Sleep _____ hours From _____ to _____

Quality of sleep _____

Exercise _____ hours From _____ to _____

Type _____

Relaxation _____ minutes From _____ to _____

Type _____

Meal	Time	Notes/Symptoms
Breakfast		
Morning Snack		
Lunch		
Afternoon Snack		
Dinner		
Medication		
Supplements		
Total glasses of water		
Bowel Movements		

Gratitude Affirmation

I am grateful for my family

Date: ___/___/___

Sleep _____ hours From _____ to _____

Quality of sleep _____

Exercise _____ hours From _____ to _____

Type _____

Relaxation _____ minutes From _____ to _____

Type_____

Meal	Time	Notes/Symptoms
Breakfast		
Morning Snack		
Lunch		
Afternoon Snack		
Dinner		
Medication		
Supplements		
Total glasses of water		
Bowel Movements		

Date: ___/___/___

Sleep _____ hours From _____ to _____

Quality of sleep _____

Exercise _____ hours From _____ to _____

Type _____

Relaxation _____ minutes From _____ to _____

Type _____

Meal	Time	Notes/Symptoms
Breakfast		
Morning Snack		
Lunch		
Afternoon Snack		
Dinner		
Medication		
Supplements		
Total glasses of water		
Bowel Movements		

Personal Challenge

Don't lie for a week.

Date: ___/___/___

Sleep   _____ hours   From _____ to _____

Quality of sleep _____

Exercise   _____ hours   From _____ to _____

Type _____

Relaxation   _____ minutes   From _____ to _____

Type _____

Meal	Time	Notes/Symptoms
Breakfast		
Morning Snack		
Lunch		
Afternoon Snack		
Dinner		
Medication		
Supplements		
Total glasses of water		
Bowel Movements		

Quote

"Sometimes there is a 36-piece orchestra going off in my stomach."
Willie Nelson

Date: ___ / ___ / ___

Sleep   _____ hours   From _____ to _____

Quality of sleep _____

Exercise   _____ hours   From _____ to _____

Type _____

Relaxation   _____ minutes   From _____ to _____

Type_____

Meal	Time	Notes/Symptoms
Breakfast		
Morning Snack		
Lunch		
Afternoon Snack		
Dinner		
Medication		
Supplements		
Total glasses of water		
Bowel Movements		

Gratitude Affirmation

I am grateful for the sun as it warms my skin and brightens my life.

Date: ___/___/___

Sleep   _____ hours   From _____ to _____

          Quality of sleep _____

Exercise   _____ hours   From _____ to _____

       Type _____

Relaxation   _____ minutes   From _____ to _____

       Type_____

Meal	Time	Notes/Symptoms
Breakfast		
Morning Snack		
Lunch		
Afternoon Snack		
Dinner		
Medication		
Supplements		
Total glasses of water		
Bowel Movements		

Health Tip

Blueberries contain resveratrol – an antioxidant compound found in red wine that is believed to help protect against heart disease and cancer.

Date: ___/___/___

Sleep _____ hours   From _____ to _____

Quality of sleep _____

Exercise _____ hours   From _____ to _____

Type _____

Relaxation _____ minutes   From _____ to _____

Type_____

Meal	Time	Notes/Symptoms
Breakfast		
Morning Snack		
Lunch		
Afternoon Snack		
Dinner		
Medication		
Supplements		
Total glasses of water		
Bowel Movements		

Personal Challenge

Say yes to everything today.
Within reason.

Date: ___/___/___

Sleep   _____ hours   From _____ to _____

Quality of sleep _____

Exercise   _____ hours   From _____ to _____

Type _____

Relaxation   _____ minutes   From _____ to _____

Type_____

Meal	Time	Notes/Symptoms
Breakfast		
Morning Snack		
Lunch		
Afternoon Snack		
Dinner		
Medication		
Supplements		
Total glasses of water		
Bowel Movements		

Date: ___ / ___ / ___

Sleep _____ hours From _____ to _____

Quality of sleep _____

Exercise _____ hours From _____ to _____

Type _____

Relaxation _____ minutes From _____ to _____

Type_____

Meal	Time	Notes/Symptoms
Breakfast		
Morning Snack		
Lunch		
Afternoon Snack		
Dinner		
Medication		
Supplements		
Total glasses of water		
Bowel Movements		

Gratitude Affirmation

I am grateful for the rain because it makes the plants that feed us grow.

Date: ___/___/___

Sleep _____ hours   From _____ to _____

Quality of sleep _____

Exercise _____ hours   From _____ to _____

Type _____

Relaxation _____ minutes   From _____ to _____

Type_____

Meal	Time	Notes/Symptoms
Breakfast		
Morning Snack		
Lunch		
Afternoon Snack		
Dinner		
Medication		
Supplements		
Total glasses of water		
Bowel Movements		

Health Tip

Folic acid can help with cancer prevention. It is found in green leafy vegetables, liver and fruit.

Date: ___/___/___

Sleep   _____ hours   From _____ to _____

Quality of sleep _____

Exercise   _____ hours   From _____ to _____

Type _____

Relaxation   _____ minutes   From _____ to _____

Type_____

Meal	Time	Notes/Symptoms
Breakfast		
Morning Snack		
Lunch		
Afternoon Snack		
Dinner		
Medication		
Supplements		
Total glasses of water		
Bowel Movements		

Personal Challenge

Let someone else be right today.

Date: ___/___/___

Sleep   _____ hours   From _____ to _____

             Quality of sleep _____

Exercise   _____ hours   From _____ to _____

      Type _____

Relaxation   _____ minutes   From _____ to _____

      Type_____

Meal	Time	Notes/Symptoms
Breakfast		
Morning Snack		
Lunch		
Afternoon Snack		
Dinner		
Medication		
Supplements		
Total glasses of water		
Bowel Movements		

Date: ___/___/___

Sleep _____ hours From _____ to _____

Quality of sleep _____

Exercise _____ hours From _____ to _____

Type _____

Relaxation _____ minutes From _____ to _____

Type_____

Meal	Time	Notes/Symptoms
Breakfast		
Morning Snack		
Lunch		
Afternoon Snack		
Dinner		
Medication		
Supplements		
Total glasses of water		
Bowel Movements		

Gratitude Affirmation

At the close of every day, I count my blessings and give thanks for all that I have.

Date: ___/___/___

Sleep   _____ hours   From _____ to _____

Quality of sleep _____

Exercise   _____ hours   From _____ to _____

Type _____

Relaxation   _____ minutes   From _____ to _____

Type _____

Meal	Time	Notes/Symptoms
Breakfast		
Morning Snack		
Lunch		
Afternoon Snack		
Dinner		
Medication		
Supplements		
Total glasses of water		
Bowel Movements		

Health Tip

Get out of the bus a stop early and walk the extra distance to work each day.

Date: ___ / ___ / ___

Sleep _____ hours From _____ to _____

Quality of sleep _____

Exercise _____ hours From _____ to _____

Type _____

Relaxation _____ minutes From _____ to _____

Type _____

Meal	Time	Notes/Symptoms
Breakfast		
Morning Snack		
Lunch		
Afternoon Snack		
Dinner		
Medication		
Supplements		
Total glasses of water		
Bowel Movements		

Personal Challenge

Give a stranger a compliment.

Date: ___/___/___

Sleep   _____ hours   From _____ to _____

Quality of sleep _____

Exercise   _____ hours   From _____ to _____

Type _____

Relaxation   _____ minutes   From _____ to _____

Type_____

Meal	Time	Notes/Symptoms
Breakfast		
Morning Snack		
Lunch		
Afternoon Snack		
Dinner		
Medication		
Supplements		
Total glasses of water		
Bowel Movements		

Date: ___/___/___

Sleep _____ hours   From _____ to _____

Quality of sleep _____

Exercise _____ hours   From _____ to _____

Type _____

Relaxation _____ minutes   From _____ to _____

Type_____

Meal	Time	Notes/Symptoms
Breakfast		
Morning Snack		
Lunch		
Afternoon Snack		
Dinner		
Medication		
Supplements		
Total glasses of water		
Bowel Movements		

I am eternally grateful for all the pleasure my senses bring me.

Date: ___/___/___

Sleep _____ hours From _____ to _____

Quality of sleep _____

Exercise _____ hours From _____ to _____

Type _____

Relaxation _____ minutes From _____ to _____

Type _____

Meal	Time	Notes/Symptoms
Breakfast		
Morning Snack		
Lunch		
Afternoon Snack		
Dinner		
Medication		
Supplements		
Total glasses of water		
Bowel Movements		

Date: ___/___/___

Sleep _____ hours From _____ to _____

Quality of sleep _____

Exercise _____ hours From _____ to _____

Type _____

Relaxation _____ minutes From _____ to _____

Type_____

Meal	Time	Notes/Symptoms
Breakfast		
Morning Snack		
Lunch		
Afternoon Snack		
Dinner		
Medication		
Supplements		
Total glasses of water		
Bowel Movements		

Personal Challenge

Go to bed at the same time each night for two weeks.

Date: ___/___/___

Sleep   _____ hours   From _____ to _____

Quality of sleep _____

Exercise   _____ hours   From _____ to _____

Type _____

Relaxation   _____ minutes   From _____ to _____

Type_____

Meal	Time	Notes/Symptoms
Breakfast		
Morning Snack		
Lunch		
Afternoon Snack		
Dinner		
Medication		
Supplements		
Total glasses of water		
Bowel Movements		

Date: ___/___/___

Sleep   _____ hours   From _____ to _____

Quality of sleep _____

Exercise   _____ hours   From _____ to _____

Type _____

Relaxation   _____ minutes   From _____ to _____

Type _____

Meal	Time	Notes/Symptoms
Breakfast		
Morning Snack		
Lunch		
Afternoon Snack		
Dinner		
Medication		
Supplements		
Total glasses of water		
Bowel Movements		

Gratitude Affirmation

I am deeply grateful for each experience life brings me.

Date: ___/___/___

Sleep   _____ hours   From _____ to _____

            Quality of sleep _____

Exercise   _____ hours   From _____ to _____

        Type _____

Relaxation   _____ minutes   From _____ to _____

        Type_____

Meal	Time	Notes/Symptoms
Breakfast		
Morning Snack		
Lunch		
Afternoon Snack		
Dinner		
Medication		
Supplements		
Total glasses of water		
Bowel Movements		

Date: ___/___/___

Sleep   _____ hours   From _____ to _____

Quality of sleep _____

Exercise   _____ hours   From _____ to _____

Type _____

Relaxation   _____ minutes   From _____ to _____

Type _____

Meal	Time	Notes/Symptoms
Breakfast		
Morning Snack		
Lunch		
Afternoon Snack		
Dinner		
Medication		
Supplements		
Total glasses of water		
Bowel Movements		

Date: ___/___/___

Sleep _____ hours   From _____ to _____

Quality of sleep _____

Exercise _____ hours   From _____ to _____

Type _____

Relaxation _____ minutes   From _____ to _____

Type _____

Meal	Time	Notes/Symptoms
Breakfast		
Morning Snack		
Lunch		
Afternoon Snack		
Dinner		
Medication		
Supplements		
Total glasses of water		
Bowel Movements		

Date: ___/___/___

Sleep   _____ hours   From _____ to _____

     Quality of sleep _____

Exercise   _____ hours   From _____ to _____

     Type _____

Relaxation   _____ minutes   From _____ to _____

     Type_____

Meal	Time	Notes/Symptoms
Breakfast		
Morning Snack		
Lunch		
Afternoon Snack		
Dinner		
Medication		
Supplements		
Total glasses of water		
Bowel Movements		

Gratitude Affirmation

I accept all gifts graciously and with deep gratitude.

Date: ___/___/___

Sleep _____ hours   From _____ to _____

Quality of sleep _____

Exercise _____ hours   From _____ to _____

Type _____

Relaxation _____ minutes   From _____ to _____

Type _____

Meal	Time	Notes/Symptoms
Breakfast		
Morning Snack		
Lunch		
Afternoon Snack		
Dinner		
Medication		
Supplements		
Total glasses of water		
Bowel Movements		

Date: ___/___/___

Sleep   _____ hours   From _____ to _____

Quality of sleep _____

Exercise   _____ hours   From _____ to _____

Type _____

Relaxation   _____ minutes   From _____ to _____

Type_____

Meal	Time	Notes/Symptoms
Breakfast		
Morning Snack		
Lunch		
Afternoon Snack		
Dinner		
Medication		
Supplements		
Total glasses of water		
Bowel Movements		

Personal Challenge

Leave your cell phone at home today.

Date: ___/___/___

Sleep   _____ hours   From _____ to _____

Quality of sleep _____

Exercise   _____ hours   From _____ to _____

Type _____

Relaxation   _____ minutes   From _____ to _____

Type_____

Meal	Time	Notes/Symptoms
Breakfast		
Morning Snack		
Lunch		
Afternoon Snack		
Dinner		
Medication		
Supplements		
Total glasses of water		
Bowel Movements		

Date: ___/___/___

Sleep   _____ hours   From _____ to _____

Quality of sleep _____

Exercise   _____ hours   From _____ to _____

Type _____

Relaxation   _____ minutes   From _____ to _____

Type _____

Meal	Time	Notes/Symptoms
Breakfast		
Morning Snack		
Lunch		
Afternoon Snack		
Dinner		
Medication		
Supplements		
Total glasses of water		
Bowel Movements		

Gratitude Affirmation

My needs and desires are generously met. For this I am thankful.

Date: ___/___/___

Sleep   _____ hours   From _____ to _____

Quality of sleep _____

Exercise   _____ hours   From _____ to _____

Type _____

Relaxation   _____ minutes   From _____ to _____

Type_____

Meal	Time	Notes/Symptoms
Breakfast		
Morning Snack		
Lunch		
Afternoon Snack		
Dinner		
Medication		
Supplements		
Total glasses of water		
Bowel Movements		

Date: ___ / ___ / ___

Sleep   _____ hours   From _____ to _____

Quality of sleep _____

Exercise   _____ hours   From _____ to _____

Type _____

Relaxation   _____ minutes   From _____ to _____

Type_____

Meal	Time	Notes/Symptoms
Breakfast		
Morning Snack		
Lunch		
Afternoon Snack		
Dinner		
Medication		
Supplements		
Total glasses of water		
Bowel Movements		

Personal Challenge

Go for a walk in the park or on the beach alone.

Date: ___/___/___

Sleep   _____ hours   From _____ to _____

Quality of sleep _____

Exercise   _____ hours   From _____ to _____

Type _____

Relaxation   _____ minutes   From _____ to _____

Type_____

Meal	Time	Notes/Symptoms
Breakfast		
Morning Snack		
Lunch		
Afternoon Snack		
Dinner		
Medication		
Supplements		
Total glasses of water		
Bowel Movements		

Date: ___/___/___

Sleep _____ hours   From _____ to _____

Quality of sleep _____

Exercise _____ hours   From _____ to _____

Type _____

Relaxation _____ minutes   From _____ to _____

Type_____

Meal	Time	Notes/Symptoms
Breakfast		
Morning Snack		
Lunch		
Afternoon Snack		
Dinner		
Medication		
Supplements		
Total glasses of water		
Bowel Movements		

Gratitude Affirmation

My mind is always effortlessly focused on positivity and thankfulness

Date: ___ / ___ / ___

Sleep _____ hours   From _____ to _____

Quality of sleep _____

Exercise _____ hours   From _____ to _____

Type _____

Relaxation _____ minutes   From _____ to _____

Type_____

Meal	Time	Notes/Symptoms
Breakfast		
Morning Snack		
Lunch		
Afternoon Snack		
Dinner		
Medication		
Supplements		
Total glasses of water		
Bowel Movements		

Health Tip

Your favourite drink has to be water. It contains no Fodmaps unlike almost every other drink.

Date: ___/___/___

Sleep _____ hours   From _____ to _____

Quality of sleep _____

Exercise _____ hours   From _____ to _____

Type _____

Relaxation _____ minutes   From _____ to _____

Type _____

Meal	Time	Notes/Symptoms
Breakfast		
Morning Snack		
Lunch		
Afternoon Snack		
Dinner		
Medication		
Supplements		
Total glasses of water		
Bowel Movements		

Sleep _____ hours From _____ to _____

Quality of sleep _____

Exercise _____ hours From _____ to _____

Type _____

Relaxation _____ minutes From _____ to _____

Type_____

Meal	Time	Notes/Symptoms
Breakfast		
Morning Snack		
Lunch		
Afternoon Snack		
Dinner		
Medication		
Supplements		
Total glasses of water		
Bowel Movements		

Date: ___/___/___

Sleep _____ hours   From _____ to _____

Quality of sleep _____

Exercise _____ hours   From _____ to _____

Type _____

Relaxation _____ minutes   From _____ to _____

Type_____

Meal	Time	Notes/Symptoms
Breakfast		
Morning Snack		
Lunch		
Afternoon Snack		
Dinner		
Medication		
Supplements		
Total glasses of water		
Bowel Movements		

Gratitude Affirmation

I am grateful for the soft bed I sleep in each night.

Date: ___/___/___

Sleep _____ hours   From _____ to _____

Quality of sleep _____

Exercise _____ hours   From _____ to _____

Type _____

Relaxation _____ minutes   From _____ to _____

Type _____

Meal	Time	Notes/Symptoms
Breakfast		
Morning Snack		
Lunch		
Afternoon Snack		
Dinner		
Medication		
Supplements		
Total glasses of water		
Bowel Movements		

Health Tip

Avoid processed foods. Check all labels and if you don't recognize all ingredients as food, put it back on the shelf. Eat as close to the source of the food as possible.

Date: ___/___/___

Sleep _____ hours   From _____ to _____

Quality of sleep _____

Exercise _____ hours   From _____ to _____

Type _____

Relaxation _____ minutes   From _____ to _____

Type_____

Meal	Time	Notes/Symptoms
Breakfast		
Morning Snack		
Lunch		
Afternoon Snack		
Dinner		
Medication		
Supplements		
Total glasses of water		
Bowel Movements		

Personal Challenge

Buy a small gift for yourself.

Date: ___/___/___

Sleep   _____ hours   From _____ to _____

Quality of sleep _____

Exercise   _____ hours   From _____ to _____

Type _____

Relaxation   _____ minutes   From _____ to _____

Type _____

Meal	Time	Notes/Symptoms
Breakfast		
Morning Snack		
Lunch		
Afternoon Snack		
Dinner		
Medication		
Supplements		
Total glasses of water		
Bowel Movements		

Date: ___/___/___

Sleep   _____ hours   From _____ to _____

                           Quality of sleep _____

Exercise   _____ hours   From _____ to _____

                Type _____

Relaxation   _____ minutes   From _____ to _____

                Type_____

Meal	Time	Notes/Symptoms
Breakfast		
Morning Snack		
Lunch		
Afternoon Snack		
Dinner		
Medication		
Supplements		
Total glasses of water		
Bowel Movements		

Gratitude Affirmation
Gratitude brings me into a harmonious relationship with the good in everyone that surrounds me.

Date: ___/___/___

Sleep _____ hours   From _____ to _____

Quality of sleep _____

Exercise _____ hours   From _____ to _____

Type _____

Relaxation _____ minutes   From _____ to _____

Type_____

Meal	Time	Notes/Symptoms
Breakfast		
Morning Snack		
Lunch		
Afternoon Snack		
Dinner		
Medication		
Supplements		
Total glasses of water		
Bowel Movements		

Date: ___/___/___

Sleep   _____ hours   From _____ to _____

Quality of sleep _____

Exercise   _____ hours   From _____ to _____

Type _____

Relaxation   _____ minutes   From _____ to _____

Type _____

Meal	Time	Notes/Symptoms
Breakfast		
Morning Snack		
Lunch		
Afternoon Snack		
Dinner		
Medication		
Supplements		
Total glasses of water		
Bowel Movements		

Personal Challenge

Write all your bad memories on paper, burn this paper afterwards. Let go.

Date: ___/___/___

Sleep _____ hours   From _____ to _____

Quality of sleep _____

Exercise _____ hours   From _____ to _____

Type _____

Relaxation _____ minutes   From _____ to _____

Type_____

Meal	Time	Notes/Symptoms
Breakfast		
Morning Snack		
Lunch		
Afternoon Snack		
Dinner		
Medication		
Supplements		
Total glasses of water		
Bowel Movements		

"*To enjoy the glow of good health, you must exercise.*"

Gene Tunney

Date: ___/___/___

Sleep _____ hours   From _____ to _____

Quality of sleep _____

Exercise _____ hours   From _____ to _____

Type _____

Relaxation _____ minutes   From _____ to _____

Type_____

Meal	Time	Notes/Symptoms
Breakfast		
Morning Snack		
Lunch		
Afternoon Snack		
Dinner		
Medication		
Supplements		
Total glasses of water		
Bowel Movements		

Gratitude Affirmation

Every day I say Thank You for what I want to see more of in my life.

Date: ___/___/___

Sleep _____ hours   From _____ to _____

Quality of sleep _____

Exercise _____ hours   From _____ to _____

Type _____

Relaxation _____ minutes   From _____ to _____

Type _____

Meal	Time	Notes/Symptoms
Breakfast		
Morning Snack		
Lunch		
Afternoon Snack		
Dinner		
Medication		
Supplements		
Total glasses of water		
Bowel Movements		

Health Tip

Balance looking after others with some self-love or you will get run down and burnt out. That kind of neglect will have a negative effect on your gut.

Date: ___/___/___

Sleep _____ hours   From _____ to _____

Quality of sleep _____

Exercise _____ hours   From _____ to _____

Type _____

Relaxation _____ minutes   From _____ to _____

Type_____

Meal	Time	Notes/Symptoms
Breakfast		
Morning Snack		
Lunch		
Afternoon Snack		
Dinner		
Medication		
Supplements		
Total glasses of water		
Bowel Movements		

Personal Challenge

Avoid elevators and escalators.
Take the stairs instead.

Date: ___/___/___

Sleep _____ hours   From _____ to _____

Quality of sleep _____

Exercise _____ hours   From _____ to _____

Type _____

Relaxation _____ minutes   From _____ to _____

Type_____

Meal	Time	Notes/Symptoms
Breakfast		
Morning Snack		
Lunch		
Afternoon Snack		
Dinner		
Medication		
Supplements		
Total glasses of water		
Bowel Movements		

Date: ___/___/___

Sleep   _____ hours   From _____ to _____

                    Quality of sleep _____

Exercise   _____ hours   From _____ to _____

            Type _____

Relaxation   _____ minutes   From _____ to _____

            Type_____

Meal	Time	Notes/Symptoms
Breakfast		
Morning Snack		
Lunch		
Afternoon Snack		
Dinner		
Medication		
Supplements		
Total glasses of water		
Bowel Movements		

Gratitude Affirmation

I am grateful for all the teachers in my life.

Date: ___/___/___

Sleep _____ hours   From _____ to _____

Quality of sleep _____

Exercise _____ hours   From _____ to _____

Type _____

Relaxation _____ minutes   From _____ to _____

Type_____

Meal	Time	Notes/Symptoms
Breakfast		
Morning Snack		
Lunch		
Afternoon Snack		
Dinner		
Medication		
Supplements		
Total glasses of water		
Bowel Movements		

Health Tip

Tomatoes contain lycopene, a powerful cancer fighter. They're also rich in vitamin C. Cooked tomatoes are also nutritious, so use them in pasta, casseroles and salads.

Date: ___/___/___

Sleep _____ hours   From _____ to _____

Quality of sleep _____

Exercise _____ hours   From _____ to _____

Type _____

Relaxation _____ minutes   From _____ to _____

Type_____

Meal	Time	Notes/Symptoms
Breakfast		
Morning Snack		
Lunch		
Afternoon Snack		
Dinner		
Medication		
Supplements		
Total glasses of water		
Bowel Movements		

Personal Challenge

Get something you have been struggling with for a while off your chest. Talk to someone you trust.

Date: ___ / ___ / ___

Sleep   _____ hours   From _____ to _____

              Quality of sleep _____

Exercise   _____ hours   From _____ to _____

       Type _____

Relaxation   _____ minutes   From _____ to _____

       Type_____

Meal	Time	Notes/Symptoms
Breakfast		
Morning Snack		
Lunch		
Afternoon Snack		
Dinner		
Medication		
Supplements		
Total glasses of water		
Bowel Movements		

Date: ___/___/___

Sleep   _____ hours   From _____ to _____

            Quality of sleep _____

Exercise   _____ hours   From _____ to _____

         Type _____

Relaxation   _____ minutes   From _____ to _____

         Type_____

Meal	Time	Notes/Symptoms
Breakfast		
Morning Snack		
Lunch		
Afternoon Snack		
Dinner		
Medication		
Supplements		
Total glasses of water		
Bowel Movements		

Gratitude Affirmation

*I am grateful for every moment that
I spend in silence.*

Date: ___ / ___ / ___

Sleep _____ hours From _____ to _____

Quality of sleep _____

Exercise _____ hours From _____ to _____

Type _____

Relaxation _____ minutes From _____ to _____

Type_____

Meal	Time	Notes/Symptoms
Breakfast		
Morning Snack		
Lunch		
Afternoon Snack		
Dinner		
Medication		
Supplements		
Total glasses of water		
Bowel Movements		

Health Tip
Mindful living - by slowing down and concentrating on basic things, you'll clear your mind of everything that worries you.

Date: ___/___/___

Sleep _____ hours   From _____ to _____

Quality of sleep _____

Exercise _____ hours   From _____ to _____

Type _____

Relaxation _____ minutes   From _____ to _____

Type_____

Meal	Time	Notes/Symptoms
Breakfast		
Morning Snack		
Lunch		
Afternoon Snack		
Dinner		
Medication		
Supplements		
Total glasses of water		
Bowel Movements		

Personal Challenge

Go see a family member you have been meaning to see

Date: ___/___/___

Sleep _____ hours   From _____ to _____

Quality of sleep _____

Exercise _____ hours   From _____ to _____

Type _____

Relaxation _____ minutes   From _____ to _____

Type_____

Meal	Time	Notes/Symptoms
Breakfast		
Morning Snack		
Lunch		
Afternoon Snack		
Dinner		
Medication		
Supplements		
Total glasses of water		
Bowel Movements		

"A fit, healthy body-- that is the best fashion statement."
Jess C. Scott

Date: ___/___/___

Sleep   _____ hours   From _____ to _____

                    Quality of sleep _____

Exercise   _____ hours   From _____ to _____

          Type _____

Relaxation   _____ minutes   From _____ to _____

          Type_____

Meal	Time	Notes/Symptoms
Breakfast		
Morning Snack		
Lunch		
Afternoon Snack		
Dinner		
Medication		
Supplements		
Total glasses of water		
Bowel Movements		

Gratitude Affirmation

I appreciate everything I have and I show my sincerest gratitude to my loved ones.

Date: ___/___/___

Sleep _____ hours From _____ to _____

Quality of sleep _____

Exercise _____ hours From _____ to _____

Type _____

Relaxation _____ minutes From _____ to _____

Type_____

Meal	Time	Notes/Symptoms
Breakfast		
Morning Snack		
Lunch		
Afternoon Snack		
Dinner		
Medication		
Supplements		
Total glasses of water		
Bowel Movements		

Health Tip

Do your weights workout before your cardio. The cardio increases blood flow to the muscles, flushing out lactic acid, which builds up in the muscles while you're weight training.

Date: ___ / ___ / ___

Sleep   _____ hours   From _____ to _____

                           Quality of sleep _____

Exercise   _____ hours   From _____ to _____

                 Type _____

Relaxation   _____ minutes   From _____ to _____

                 Type_____

Meal	Time	Notes/Symptoms
Breakfast		
Morning Snack		
Lunch		
Afternoon Snack		
Dinner		
Medication		
Supplements		
Total glasses of water		
Bowel Movements		

Personal Challenge

Smile at yourself in the mirror for at least 10 seconds.

Date: ___/___/___

Sleep   _____ hours   From _____ to _____

         Quality of sleep _____

Exercise   _____ hours   From _____ to _____

       Type _____

Relaxation   _____ minutes   From _____ to _____

       Type_____

Meal	Time	Notes/Symptoms
Breakfast		
Morning Snack		
Lunch		
Afternoon Snack		
Dinner		
Medication		
Supplements		
Total glasses of water		
Bowel Movements		

Date: ___/___/___

Sleep _____ hours   From _____ to _____

Quality of sleep _____

Exercise _____ hours   From _____ to _____

Type _____

Relaxation _____ minutes   From _____ to _____

Type _____

Meal	Time	Notes/Symptoms
Breakfast		
Morning Snack		
Lunch		
Afternoon Snack		
Dinner		
Medication		
Supplements		
Total glasses of water		
Bowel Movements		

Gratitude Affirmation

I clearly see the beauty of life that flourishes around me.

Date: ___/___/___

Sleep _____ hours   From _____ to _____

Quality of sleep _____

Exercise _____ hours   From _____ to _____

Type _____

Relaxation _____ minutes   From _____ to _____

Type_____

Meal	Time	Notes/Symptoms
Breakfast		
Morning Snack		
Lunch		
Afternoon Snack		
Dinner		
Medication		
Supplements		
Total glasses of water		
Bowel Movements		

Health Tip

IBS is connected to hormonal fluctuations so women will feel their cycles more acutely than someone without IBS.

Date: ___/___/___

Sleep   _____ hours   From _____ to _____

                 Quality of sleep _____

Exercise   _____ hours   From _____ to _____

           Type _____

Relaxation   _____ minutes   From _____ to _____

           Type_____

Meal	Time	Notes/Symptoms
Breakfast		
Morning Snack		
Lunch		
Afternoon Snack		
Dinner		
Medication		
Supplements		
Total glasses of water		
Bowel Movements		

Personal Challenge

Pick up a piece of litter and place it in a bin. If we all did that every day, our streets would be

Date: ___ / ___ / ___

Sleep   _____ hours   From _____ to _____

Quality of sleep _____

Exercise   _____ hours   From _____ to _____

Type _____

Relaxation   _____ minutes   From _____ to _____

Type_____

Meal	Time	Notes/Symptoms
Breakfast		
Morning Snack		
Lunch		
Afternoon Snack		
Dinner		
Medication		
Supplements		
Total glasses of water		
Bowel Movements		

Date: _____/_____/_____

Sleep   _____ hours   From _____ to _____

Quality of sleep _____

Exercise   _____ hours   From _____ to _____

Type _____

Relaxation   _____ minutes   From _____ to _____

Type_____

Meal	Time	Notes/Symptoms
Breakfast		
Morning Snack		
Lunch		
Afternoon Snack		
Dinner		
Medication		
Supplements		
Total glasses of water		
Bowel Movements		

Gratitude Affirmation

My thoughts are focused on positivity and thankfulness

Date: ___ / ___ / ___

Sleep _____ hours   From _____ to _____

Quality of sleep _____

Exercise _____ hours   From _____ to _____

Type _____

Relaxation _____ minutes   From _____ to _____

Type_____

Meal	Time	Notes/Symptoms
Breakfast		
Morning Snack		
Lunch		
Afternoon Snack		
Dinner		
Medication		
Supplements		
Total glasses of water		
Bowel Movements		

Health Tip

Make sure you get enough vitamin C to keep your immune system strong. Eat citrus fruits, kiwifruit , tomatoes, papaya and red peppers.

Date: ___ / ___ / ___

Sleep _____ hours   From _____ to _____

Quality of sleep _____

Exercise _____ hours   From _____ to _____

Type _____

Relaxation _____ minutes   From _____ to _____

Type _____

Meal	Time	Notes/Symptoms
Breakfast		
Morning Snack		
Lunch		
Afternoon Snack		
Dinner		
Medication		
Supplements		
Total glasses of water		
Bowel Movements		

Personal Challenge

Don't say anything negative today.
Focus on the positive.

Date: ___/___/___

Sleep   _____ hours   From _____ to _____

            Quality of sleep _____

Exercise   _____ hours   From _____ to _____

            Type _____

Relaxation   _____ minutes   From _____ to _____

            Type_____

Meal	Time	Notes/Symptoms
Breakfast		
Morning Snack		
Lunch		
Afternoon Snack		
Dinner		
Medication		
Supplements		
Total glasses of water		
Bowel Movements		

Date: ___/___/___

Sleep _____ hours From _____ to _____

Quality of sleep _____

Exercise _____ hours From _____ to _____

Type _____

Relaxation _____ minutes From _____ to _____

Type _____

Meal	Time	Notes/Symptoms
Breakfast		
Morning Snack		
Lunch		
Afternoon Snack		
Dinner		
Medication		
Supplements		
Total glasses of water		
Bowel Movements		

Gratitude Affirmation

I give thanks continually as I move through each day.

Date: ___/___/___

Sleep   _____ hours   From _____ to _____

Quality of sleep _____

Exercise   _____ hours   From _____ to _____

Type _____

Relaxation   _____ minutes   From _____ to _____

Type_____

Meal	Time	Notes/Symptoms
Breakfast		
Morning Snack		
Lunch		
Afternoon Snack		
Dinner		
Medication		
Supplements		
Total glasses of water		
Bowel Movements		

Health Tip

Hunger is the enemy of someone with IBS so always keep low Fodmap snacks on hand in case you get held up somewhere without low Fodmap food when your next meal time arrives.

Date: ___ / ___ / ___

Sleep   _____ hours   From _____ to _____

                  Quality of sleep _____

Exercise   _____ hours   From _____ to _____

         Type _____

Relaxation   _____ minutes   From _____ to _____

         Type_____

Meal	Time	Notes/Symptoms
Breakfast		
Morning Snack		
Lunch		
Afternoon Snack		
Dinner		
Medication		
Supplements		
Total glasses of water		
Bowel Movements		

Date: ___/___/___

Sleep   _____ hours   From _____ to _____

Quality of sleep _____

Exercise   _____ hours   From _____ to _____

Type _____

Relaxation   _____ minutes   From _____ to _____

Type_____

Meal	Time	Notes/Symptoms
Breakfast		
Morning Snack		
Lunch		
Afternoon Snack		
Dinner		
Medication		
Supplements		
Total glasses of water		
Bowel Movements		

Date: ___/___/___

Sleep _____ hours   From _____ to _____

Quality of sleep _____

Exercise _____ hours   From _____ to _____

Type _____

Relaxation _____ minutes   From _____ to _____

Type_____

Meal	Time	Notes/Symptoms
Breakfast		
Morning Snack		
Lunch		
Afternoon Snack		
Dinner		
Medication		
Supplements		
Total glasses of water		
Bowel Movements		

Gratitude Affirmation

An attitude of gratitude is the key to manifesting a better life for myself.

Date: ___/___/___

Sleep   _____ hours   From _____ to _____

            Quality of sleep _____

Exercise   _____ hours   From _____ to _____

            Type _____

Relaxation   _____ minutes   From _____ to _____

            Type_____

Meal	Time	Notes/Symptoms
Breakfast		
Morning Snack		
Lunch		
Afternoon Snack		
Dinner		
Medication		
Supplements		
Total glasses of water		
Bowel Movements		

Health Tip

If you have reflux, avoid tomatoes, citrus fruits, spicy food, oily food, caffeine, mint and alcohol. Also don't lie down after eating, and eat at least 3 hours before bed.

Date: ___/___/___

Sleep   _____ hours   From _____ to _____

Quality of sleep _____

Exercise   _____ hours   From _____ to _____

Type _____

Relaxation   _____ minutes   From _____ to _____

Type _____

Meal	Time	Notes/Symptoms
Breakfast		
Morning Snack		
Lunch		
Afternoon Snack		
Dinner		
Medication		
Supplements		
Total glasses of water		
Bowel Movements		

Personal Challenge

Spend a few minutes deleting unnecessary contacts from your phone.

Date: ___/___/___

Sleep   _____ hours   From _____ to _____

Quality of sleep _____

Exercise   _____ hours   From _____ to _____

Type _____

Relaxation   _____ minutes   From _____ to _____

Type_____

Meal	Time	Notes/Symptoms
Breakfast		
Morning Snack		
Lunch		
Afternoon Snack		
Dinner		
Medication		
Supplements		
Total glasses of water		
Bowel Movements		

Date:___/___/___

Sleep _____ hours   From _____ to _____

Quality of sleep _____

Exercise _____ hours   From _____ to _____

Type _____

Relaxation _____ minutes   From _____ to _____

Type_____

Meal	Time	Notes/Symptoms
Breakfast		
Morning Snack		
Lunch		
Afternoon Snack		
Dinner		
Medication		
Supplements		
Total glasses of water		
Bowel Movements		

Gratitude Affirmation

I am grateful for my house which shelters me from the elements.

Date: ___/___/___

Sleep _____ hours   From _____ to _____

Quality of sleep _____

Exercise _____ hours   From _____ to _____

Type _____

Relaxation _____ minutes   From _____ to _____

Type_____

Meal	Time	Notes/Symptoms
Breakfast		
Morning Snack		
Lunch		
Afternoon Snack		
Dinner		
Medication		
Supplements		
Total glasses of water		
Bowel Movements		

Date: ___/___/___

Sleep   _____ hours   From _____ to _____

Quality of sleep _____

Exercise   _____ hours   From _____ to _____

Type _____

Relaxation   _____ minutes   From _____ to _____

Type _____

Meal	Time	Notes/Symptoms
Breakfast		
Morning Snack		
Lunch		
Afternoon Snack		
Dinner		
Medication		
Supplements		
Total glasses of water		
Bowel Movements		

Sleep   _____ hours   From _____ to _____

Quality of sleep _____

Exercise   _____ hours   From _____ to _____

Type _____

Relaxation   _____ minutes   From _____ to _____

Type _____

Meal	Time	Notes/Symptoms
Breakfast		
Morning Snack		
Lunch		
Afternoon Snack		
Dinner		
Medication		
Supplements		
Total glasses of water		
Bowel Movements		

Date: ___ / ___ / ___

Sleep   _____ hours   From _____ to _____

Quality of sleep _____

Exercise   _____ hours   From _____ to _____

Type _____

Relaxation   _____ minutes   From _____ to _____

Type_____

Meal	Time	Notes/Symptoms
Breakfast		
Morning Snack		
Lunch		
Afternoon Snack		
Dinner		
Medication		
Supplements		
Total glasses of water		
Bowel Movements		

Gratitude Affirmation

I am forever grateful for being able to contribute to the lives of others.

Date: ___/___/___

Sleep _____ hours   From _____ to _____

Quality of sleep _____

Exercise _____ hours   From _____ to _____

Type _____

Relaxation _____ minutes   From _____ to _____

Type_____

Meal	Time	Notes/Symptoms
Breakfast		
Morning Snack		
Lunch		
Afternoon Snack		
Dinner		
Medication		
Supplements		
Total glasses of water		
Bowel Movements		

Health Tip

For constipation, drink 8 glasses of water and exercise daily. Also make sure you have an adequate intake of fibre and fats/oil.

Date: ___/___/___

Sleep _____ hours From _____ to _____

Quality of sleep _____

Exercise _____ hours From _____ to _____

Type _____

Relaxation _____ minutes From _____ to _____

Type _____

Meal	Time	Notes/Symptoms
Breakfast		
Morning Snack		
Lunch		
Afternoon Snack		
Dinner		
Medication		
Supplements		
Total glasses of water		
Bowel Movements		

Personal Challenge

Create your own dance for your happy moments.

Date: ___/___/___

Sleep   _____ hours   From _____ to _____

                 Quality of sleep _____

Exercise   _____ hours   From _____ to _____

            Type _____

Relaxation   _____ minutes   From _____ to _____

            Type_____

Meal	Time	Notes/Symptoms
Breakfast		
Morning Snack		
Lunch		
Afternoon Snack		
Dinner		
Medication		
Supplements		
Total glasses of water		
Bowel Movements		

Date: ___/___/___

Sleep _____ hours From _____ to _____

Quality of sleep _____

Exercise _____ hours From _____ to _____

Type _____

Relaxation _____ minutes From _____ to _____

Type _____

Meal	Time	Notes/Symptoms
Breakfast		
Morning Snack		
Lunch		
Afternoon Snack		
Dinner		
Medication		
Supplements		
Total glasses of water		
Bowel Movements		

Gratitude Affirmation

I am grateful for being able to hear my intuition.

Date: ___/___/___

Sleep   _____ hours   From _____ to _____

         Quality of sleep _____

Exercise   _____ hours   From _____ to _____

         Type _____

Relaxation   _____ minutes   From _____ to _____

         Type _____

Meal	Time	Notes/Symptoms
Breakfast		
Morning Snack		
Lunch		
Afternoon Snack		
Dinner		
Medication		
Supplements		
Total glasses of water		
Bowel Movements		

Date: ___/___/___

Sleep   _____ hours   From _____ to _____

Quality of sleep _____

Exercise   _____ hours   From _____ to _____

Type _____

Relaxation   _____ minutes   From _____ to _____

Type _____

Meal	Time	Notes/Symptoms
Breakfast		
Morning Snack		
Lunch		
Afternoon Snack		
Dinner		
Medication		
Supplements		
Total glasses of water		
Bowel Movements		

Date: ___/___/___

Sleep   _____ hours   From _____ to _____

Quality of sleep _____

Exercise   _____ hours   From _____ to _____

Type _____

Relaxation   _____ minutes   From _____ to _____

Type _____

Meal	Time	Notes/Symptoms
Breakfast		
Morning Snack		
Lunch		
Afternoon Snack		
Dinner		
Medication		
Supplements		
Total glasses of water		
Bowel Movements		

Date: ___/___/___

Sleep _____ hours From _____ to _____

Quality of sleep _____

Exercise _____ hours From _____ to _____

Type _____

Relaxation _____ minutes From _____ to _____

Type_____

Meal	Time	Notes/Symptoms
Breakfast		
Morning Snack		
Lunch		
Afternoon Snack		
Dinner		
Medication		
Supplements		
Total glasses of water		
Bowel Movements		

Gratitude Affirmation

I am grateful for my wonderful life.

Date: ___/___/___

Sleep _____ hours From _____ to _____

Quality of sleep _____

Exercise _____ hours From _____ to _____

Type _____

Relaxation _____ minutes From _____ to _____

Type _____

Meal	Time	Notes/Symptoms
Breakfast		
Morning Snack		
Lunch		
Afternoon Snack		
Dinner		
Medication		
Supplements		
Total glasses of water		
Bowel Movements		

Date: ___/___/___

Sleep _____ hours   From _____ to _____

Quality of sleep _____

Exercise _____ hours   From _____ to _____

Type _____

Relaxation _____ minutes   From _____ to _____

Type_____

Meal	Time	Notes/Symptoms
Breakfast		
Morning Snack		
Lunch		
Afternoon Snack		
Dinner		
Medication		
Supplements		
Total glasses of water		
Bowel Movements		

Personal Challenge

Take some time to watch the sunset or sunrise.

Date: ___/___/___

Sleep   _____ hours   From _____ to _____

         Quality of sleep _____

Exercise   _____ hours   From _____ to _____

         Type _____

Relaxation   _____ minutes   From _____ to _____

         Type_____

Meal	Time	Notes/Symptoms
Breakfast		
Morning Snack		
Lunch		
Afternoon Snack		
Dinner		
Medication		
Supplements		
Total glasses of water		
Bowel Movements		

Date: ___/___/___

Sleep   _____ hours   From _____ to _____

Quality of sleep _____

Exercise   _____ hours   From _____ to _____

Type _____

Relaxation   _____ minutes   From _____ to _____

Type _____

Meal	Time	Notes/Symptoms
Breakfast		
Morning Snack		
Lunch		
Afternoon Snack		
Dinner		
Medication		
Supplements		
Total glasses of water		
Bowel Movements		

Gratitude Affirmation

I am truly grateful for the support I receive from my family and friends.

Date: ___ / ___ / ___

Sleep   _____ hours   From _____ to _____

                   Quality of sleep _____

Exercise   _____ hours   From _____ to _____

               Type _____

Relaxation   _____ minutes   From _____ to _____

               Type_____

Meal	Time	Notes/Symptoms
Breakfast		
Morning Snack		
Lunch		
Afternoon Snack		
Dinner		
Medication		
Supplements		
Total glasses of water		
Bowel Movements		

Health Tip
Add spices and herbs to your meals
to create tasty food that doesn't
make you feel deprived.

Date: ___ / ___ / ___

Sleep _____ hours   From _____ to _____

Quality of sleep _____

Exercise _____ hours   From _____ to _____

Type _____

Relaxation _____ minutes   From _____ to _____

Type_____

Meal	Time	Notes/Symptoms
Breakfast		
Morning Snack		
Lunch		
Afternoon Snack		
Dinner		
Medication		
Supplements		
Total glasses of water		
Bowel Movements		

Personal Challenge

Buy your mum or sister flowers.

Date: ___/___/___

Sleep   _____ hours   From _____ to _____

Quality of sleep _____

Exercise   _____ hours   From _____ to _____

Type _____

Relaxation   _____ minutes   From _____ to _____

Type_____

Meal	Time	Notes/Symptoms
Breakfast		
Morning Snack		
Lunch		
Afternoon Snack		
Dinner		
Medication		
Supplements		
Total glasses of water		
Bowel Movements		

Date: ___/___/___

Sleep _____ hours   From _____ to _____

Quality of sleep _____

Exercise _____ hours   From _____ to _____

Type _____

Relaxation _____ minutes   From _____ to _____

Type_____

Meal	Time	Notes/Symptoms
Breakfast		
Morning Snack		
Lunch		
Afternoon Snack		
Dinner		
Medication		
Supplements		
Total glasses of water		
Bowel Movements		

Gratitude Affirmation

I cherish each and every moment in my life.

Date: ___/___/___

Sleep   _____ hours   From _____ to _____

                     Quality of sleep _____

Exercise   _____ hours   From _____ to _____

            Type _____

Relaxation   _____ minutes   From _____ to _____

            Type_____

Meal	Time	Notes/Symptoms
Breakfast		
Morning Snack		
Lunch		
Afternoon Snack		
Dinner		
Medication		
Supplements		
Total glasses of water		
Bowel Movements		

Date: ___/___/___

Sleep _____ hours From _____ to _____

Quality of sleep _____

Exercise _____ hours From _____ to _____

Type _____

Relaxation _____ minutes From _____ to _____

Type_____

Meal	Time	Notes/Symptoms
Breakfast		
Morning Snack		
Lunch		
Afternoon Snack		
Dinner		
Medication		
Supplements		
Total glasses of water		
Bowel Movements		

Personal Challenge

Change your name for the day.

Date: ___ / ___ / ___

Sleep _____ hours   From _____ to _____

Quality of sleep _____

Exercise _____ hours   From _____ to _____

Type _____

Relaxation _____ minutes   From _____ to _____

Type _____

Meal	Time	Notes/Symptoms
Breakfast		
Morning Snack		
Lunch		
Afternoon Snack		
Dinner		
Medication		
Supplements		
Total glasses of water		
Bowel Movements		

Date: ___/___/___

Sleep _____ hours From _____ to _____

Quality of sleep _____

Exercise _____ hours From _____ to _____

Type _____

Relaxation _____ minutes From _____ to _____

Type _____

Meal	Time	Notes/Symptoms
Breakfast		
Morning Snack		
Lunch		
Afternoon Snack		
Dinner		
Medication		
Supplements		
Total glasses of water		
Bowel Movements		

Gratitude Affirmation

Thankfulness keeps me connected to universal abundance.

Date: ___/___/___

Sleep _____ hours   From _____ to _____

Quality of sleep _____

Exercise _____ hours   From _____ to _____

Type _____

Relaxation _____ minutes   From _____ to _____

Type_____

Meal	Time	Notes/Symptoms
Breakfast		
Morning Snack		
Lunch		
Afternoon Snack		
Dinner		
Medication		
Supplements		
Total glasses of water		
Bowel Movements		

Date: ___ / ___ / ___

Sleep _____ hours   From _____ to _____

Quality of sleep _____

Exercise _____ hours   From _____ to _____

Type _____

Relaxation _____ minutes   From _____ to _____

Type _____

Meal	Time	Notes/Symptoms
Breakfast		
Morning Snack		
Lunch		
Afternoon Snack		
Dinner		
Medication		
Supplements		
Total glasses of water		
Bowel Movements		

Personal Challenge

Write down at least 10 things you're grateful for and hang the sheet of paper in your room.

Date: ___/___/___

Sleep   _____ hours   From _____ to _____

          Quality of sleep _____

Exercise   _____ hours   From _____ to _____

        Type _____

Relaxation   _____ minutes   From _____ to _____

        Type_____

Meal	Time	Notes/Symptoms
Breakfast		
Morning Snack		
Lunch		
Afternoon Snack		
Dinner		
Medication		
Supplements		
Total glasses of water		
Bowel Movements		

Date: ___/___/___

Sleep _____ hours   From _____ to _____

Quality of sleep _____

Exercise _____ hours   From _____ to _____

Type _____

Relaxation _____ minutes   From _____ to _____

Type_____

Meal	Time	Notes/Symptoms
Breakfast		
Morning Snack		
Lunch		
Afternoon Snack		
Dinner		
Medication		
Supplements		
Total glasses of water		
Bowel Movements		

Gratitude Affirmation

At the end of each day, I take a moment to reflect and be grateful.

Date: ___/___/___

Sleep   _____ hours   From _____ to _____

Quality of sleep _____

Exercise   _____ hours   From _____ to _____

Type _____

Relaxation   _____ minutes   From _____ to _____

Type_____

Meal	Time	Notes/Symptoms
Breakfast		
Morning Snack		
Lunch		
Afternoon Snack		
Dinner		
Medication		
Supplements		
Total glasses of water		
Bowel Movements		

Health Tip

Make sure you get enough fibre on the low Fodmap diet but not too much because fibre is a gut irritant. Good sources are quinoa, oats, brown rice, oat and rice bran, fruit and vegetables.

Date: ___ / ___ / ___

Sleep   _____ hours   From _____ to _____

                      Quality of sleep _____

Exercise   _____ hours   From _____ to _____

            Type _____

Relaxation   _____ minutes   From _____ to _____

            Type_____

Meal	Time	Notes/Symptoms
Breakfast		
Morning Snack		
Lunch		
Afternoon Snack		
Dinner		
Medication		
Supplements		
Total glasses of water		
Bowel Movements		

Personal Challenge

Do something impulsive.

Date: ___/___/___

Sleep _____ hours   From _____ to _____

Quality of sleep _____

Exercise _____ hours   From _____ to _____

Type _____

Relaxation _____ minutes   From _____ to _____

Type_____

Meal	Time	Notes/Symptoms
Breakfast		
Morning Snack		
Lunch		
Afternoon Snack		
Dinner		
Medication		
Supplements		
Total glasses of water		
Bowel Movements		

Quote

"Be careful about reading health
books. You may die of a misprint."
Mark Twain

Date: ___/___/___

Sleep   _____ hours   From _____ to _____

                  Quality of sleep _____

Exercise   _____ hours   From _____ to _____

            Type _____

Relaxation   _____ minutes   From _____ to _____

            Type_____

Meal	Time	Notes/Symptoms
Breakfast		
Morning Snack		
Lunch		
Afternoon Snack		
Dinner		
Medication		
Supplements		
Total glasses of water		
Bowel Movements		

Gratitude Affirmation

Every day I thank the universe for showing me the way to my dreams.

Date: ___/___/___

Sleep _____ hours From _____ to _____

Quality of sleep _____

Exercise _____ hours From _____ to _____

Type _____

Relaxation _____ minutes From _____ to _____

Type _____

Meal	Time	Notes/Symptoms
Breakfast		
Morning Snack		
Lunch		
Afternoon Snack		
Dinner		
Medication		
Supplements		
Total glasses of water		
Bowel Movements		

Health Tip

A adequate iron intake is important and your needs can be met by all meats, especially red meat, shellfish and sardines. Tofu also has a decent amount of iron as do iron-enriched cereals.

Date: ___/___/___

Sleep _____ hours From _____ to _____

Quality of sleep _____

Exercise _____ hours From _____ to _____

Type _____

Relaxation _____ minutes From _____ to _____

Type _____

Meal	Time	Notes/Symptoms
Breakfast		
Morning Snack		
Lunch		
Afternoon Snack		
Dinner		
Medication		
Supplements		
Total glasses of water		
Bowel Movements		

Personal Challenge

Actively listen to someone's concerns and problems.

Date: ___/___/___

Sleep _____ hours From _____ to _____

Quality of sleep _____

Exercise _____ hours From _____ to _____

Type _____

Relaxation _____ minutes From _____ to _____

Type_____

Meal	Time	Notes/Symptoms
Breakfast		
Morning Snack		
Lunch		
Afternoon Snack		
Dinner		
Medication		
Supplements		
Total glasses of water		
Bowel Movements		

Date: ___/___/___

Sleep _____ hours   From _____ to _____

Quality of sleep _____

Exercise _____ hours   From _____ to _____

Type _____

Relaxation _____ minutes   From _____ to _____

Type_____

Meal	Time	Notes/Symptoms
Breakfast		
Morning Snack		
Lunch		
Afternoon Snack		
Dinner		
Medication		
Supplements		
Total glasses of water		
Bowel Movements		

Gratitude Affirmation

I am so grateful to be alive and well.

Date: ___/___/___

Sleep _____ hours   From _____ to _____

Quality of sleep _____

Exercise _____ hours   From _____ to _____

Type _____

Relaxation _____ minutes   From _____ to _____

Type_____

Meal	Time	Notes/Symptoms
Breakfast		
Morning Snack		
Lunch		
Afternoon Snack		
Dinner		
Medication		
Supplements		
Total glasses of water		
Bowel Movements		

Date: ___/___/___

Sleep   _____ hours   From _____ to _____

Quality of sleep _____

Exercise   _____ hours   From _____ to _____

Type _____

Relaxation   _____ minutes   From _____ to _____

Type_____

Meal	Time	Notes/Symptoms
Breakfast		
Morning Snack		
Lunch		
Afternoon Snack		
Dinner		
Medication		
Supplements		
Total glasses of water		
Bowel Movements		

Personal Challenge

Make plans to visit someone who does not live close to you.

Date: ___/___/___

Sleep _____ hours   From _____ to _____

Quality of sleep _____

Exercise _____ hours   From _____ to _____

Type _____

Relaxation _____ minutes   From _____ to _____

Type _____

Meal	Time	Notes/Symptoms
Breakfast		
Morning Snack		
Lunch		
Afternoon Snack		
Dinner		
Medication		
Supplements		
Total glasses of water		
Bowel Movements		

Quote

*"A good laugh and a long sleep are
the best cures in the doctor's book."*
Irish Proverb

Date: ___/___/___

Sleep _____ hours From _____ to _____

Quality of sleep _____

Exercise _____ hours From _____ to _____

Type _____

Relaxation _____ minutes From _____ to _____

Type_____

Meal	Time	Notes/Symptoms
Breakfast		
Morning Snack		
Lunch		
Afternoon Snack		
Dinner		
Medication		
Supplements		
Total glasses of water		
Bowel Movements		

Gratitude Affirmation

I am thankful for the trees that provide the planet with oxygen.

Date: ___/___/___

Sleep   _____ hours   From _____ to _____

                   Quality of sleep _____

Exercise   _____ hours   From _____ to _____

            Type _____

Relaxation   _____ minutes   From _____ to _____

            Type_____

Meal	Time	Notes/Symptoms
Breakfast		
Morning Snack		
Lunch		
Afternoon Snack		
Dinner		
Medication		
Supplements		
Total glasses of water		
Bowel Movements		

Health Tip

The best milk for the low Fodmap diet is either oat, rice or lactose-free. Soya milk must be made from the protein of the bean to be acceptable. Avoid almond milk until it has been tested.

Date: ___/___/___

Sleep   _____ hours   From _____ to _____

               Quality of sleep _____

Exercise   _____ hours   From _____ to _____

          Type _____

Relaxation   _____ minutes   From _____ to _____

          Type_____

Meal	Time	Notes/Symptoms
Breakfast		
Morning Snack		
Lunch		
Afternoon Snack		
Dinner		
Medication		
Supplements		
Total glasses of water		
Bowel Movements		

Personal Challenge

Loan or buy someone your favourite book.

Date: ___/___/__

Sleep   _____ hours   From _____ to _____

                 Quality of sleep _____

Exercise   _____ hours   From _____ to _____

          Type _____

Relaxation   _____ minutes   From _____ to _____

          Type_____

Meal	Time	Notes/Symptoms
Breakfast		
Morning Snack		
Lunch		
Afternoon Snack		
Dinner		
Medication		
Supplements		
Total glasses of water		
Bowel Movements		

Date: ___/___/___

Sleep   _____ hours   From _____ to _____

Quality of sleep _____

Exercise   _____ hours   From _____ to _____

Type _____

Relaxation   _____ minutes   From _____ to _____

Type_____

Meal	Time	Notes/Symptoms
Breakfast		
Morning Snack		
Lunch		
Afternoon Snack		
Dinner		
Medication		
Supplements		
Total glasses of water		
Bowel Movements		

Gratitude Affirmation

I am thankful for every spark of insight that inspires me.

Date: ___/___/___

Sleep _____ hours From _____ to _____

Quality of sleep _____

Exercise _____ hours From _____ to _____

Type _____

Relaxation _____ minutes From _____ to _____

Type_____

Meal	Time	Notes/Symptoms
Breakfast		
Morning Snack		
Lunch		
Afternoon Snack		
Dinner		
Medication		
Supplements		
Total glasses of water		
Bowel Movements		

Date: ___/___/___

Sleep   _____ hours   From _____ to _____

                Quality of sleep _____

Exercise   _____ hours   From _____ to _____

          Type _____

Relaxation   _____ minutes   From _____ to _____

          Type_____

Meal	Time	Notes/Symptoms
Breakfast		
Morning Snack		
Lunch		
Afternoon Snack		
Dinner		
Medication		
Supplements		
Total glasses of water		
Bowel Movements		

Personal Challenge

Make someone laugh today.

Date: ___/___/___

Sleep   _____ hours   From _____ to _____

                                Quality of sleep _____

Exercise   _____ hours   From _____ to _____

                         Type _____

Relaxation   _____ minutes   From _____ to _____

                         Type_____

Meal	Time	Notes/Symptoms
Breakfast		
Morning Snack		
Lunch		
Afternoon Snack		
Dinner		
Medication		
Supplements		
Total glasses of water		
Bowel Movements		

Date: ___/___/___

Sleep _____ hours From _____ to _____

Quality of sleep _____

Exercise _____ hours From _____ to _____

Type _____

Relaxation _____ minutes From _____ to _____

Type_____

Meal	Time	Notes/Symptoms
Breakfast		
Morning Snack		
Lunch		
Afternoon Snack		
Dinner		
Medication		
Supplements		
Total glasses of water		
Bowel Movements		

Gratitude Affirmation

I have a wonderful life and for that I give my unending gratitude.

Date: ___/___/___

Sleep _____ hours   From _____ to _____

Quality of sleep _____

Exercise _____ hours   From _____ to _____

Type _____

Relaxation _____ minutes   From _____ to _____

Type_____

Meal	Time	Notes/Symptoms
Breakfast		
Morning Snack		
Lunch		
Afternoon Snack		
Dinner		
Medication		
Supplements		
Total glasses of water		
Bowel Movements		

Health Tip

If you have trapped gas, try some appropriate yoga poses or other gentle exercise like walking to relax the muscles. You can also use heat in the form of a warm bath or a heat pack.

Date: ___/___/___

Sleep _____ hours From _____ to _____

Quality of sleep _____

Exercise _____ hours From _____ to _____

Type _____

Relaxation _____ minutes From _____ to _____

Type _____

Meal	Time	Notes/Symptoms
Breakfast		
Morning Snack		
Lunch		
Afternoon Snack		
Dinner		
Medication		
Supplements		
Total glasses of water		
Bowel Movements		

Personal Challenge

Get someone you love a small gift.

Date: ___/___/___

Sleep   _____ hours   From _____ to _____

          Quality of sleep _____

Exercise   _____ hours   From _____ to _____

        Type _____

Relaxation   _____ minutes   From _____ to _____

        Type_____

Meal	Time	Notes/Symptoms
Breakfast		
Morning Snack		
Lunch		
Afternoon Snack		
Dinner		
Medication		
Supplements		
Total glasses of water		
Bowel Movements		

Date: ___/___/___

Sleep _____ hours From _____ to _____

Quality of sleep _____

Exercise _____ hours From _____ to _____

Type _____

Relaxation _____ minutes From _____ to _____

Type _____

Meal	Time	Notes/Symptoms
Breakfast		
Morning Snack		
Lunch		
Afternoon Snack		
Dinner		
Medication		
Supplements		
Total glasses of water		
Bowel Movements		

Gratitude Affirmation

I take the time to appreciate the simple things in life.

Date: ___/___/___

Sleep   _____ hours   From _____ to _____

Quality of sleep _____

Exercise   _____ hours   From _____ to _____

Type _____

Relaxation   _____ minutes   From _____ to _____

Type_____

Meal	Time	Notes/Symptoms
Breakfast		
Morning Snack		
Lunch		
Afternoon Snack		
Dinner		
Medication		
Supplements		
Total glasses of water		
Bowel Movements		

Health Tip

If you do go off track on the diet and symptoms return, get straight back on the diet and expect the upset to last for up to two days. Don't give up at this stage but hang tough.

Date: ___/___/___

Sleep   _____ hours   From _____ to _____

Quality of sleep _____

Exercise   _____ hours   From _____ to _____

Type _____

Relaxation   _____ minutes   From _____ to _____

Type_____

Meal	Time	Notes/Symptoms
Breakfast		
Morning Snack		
Lunch		
Afternoon Snack		
Dinner		
Medication		
Supplements		
Total glasses of water		
Bowel Movements		

Personal Challenge

Watch your favourite movie.

Date: ___/___/___

Sleep _____ hours   From _____ to _____

Quality of sleep _____

Exercise _____ hours   From _____ to _____

Type _____

Relaxation _____ minutes   From _____ to _____

Type _____

Meal	Time	Notes/Symptoms
Breakfast		
Morning Snack		
Lunch		
Afternoon Snack		
Dinner		
Medication		
Supplements		
Total glasses of water		
Bowel Movements		

Date: ___/___/___

Sleep   _____ hours   From _____ to _____

Quality of sleep _____

Exercise   _____ hours   From _____ to _____

Type _____

Relaxation   _____ minutes   From _____ to _____

Type _____

Meal	Time	Notes/Symptoms
Breakfast		
Morning Snack		
Lunch		
Afternoon Snack		
Dinner		
Medication		
Supplements		
Total glasses of water		
Bowel Movements		

Gratitude Affirmation

Each Morning I give thanks for another day of life.

Date: ___/___/___

Sleep   _____ hours   From _____ to _____

         Quality of sleep _____

Exercise   _____ hours   From _____ to _____

       Type _____

Relaxation   _____ minutes   From _____ to _____

       Type_____

Meal	Time	Notes/Symptoms
Breakfast		
Morning Snack		
Lunch		
Afternoon Snack		
Dinner		
Medication		
Supplements		
Total glasses of water		
Bowel Movements		

Health Tip

Caffeine is a gut irritant and should be avoided as much as possible though weak tea or coffee once or twice a day should be acceptable, depending on your individual tolerance.

Date: ___/___/___

Sleep _____ hours From _____ to _____

Quality of sleep _____

Exercise _____ hours From _____ to _____

Type _____

Relaxation _____ minutes From _____ to _____

Type _____

Meal	Time	Notes/Symptoms
Breakfast		
Morning Snack		
Lunch		
Afternoon Snack		
Dinner		
Medication		
Supplements		
Total glasses of water		
Bowel Movements		

Personal Challenge

Do the thing you would do if it were your last day on earth.

Date: ___/___/___

Sleep _____ hours   From _____ to _____

Quality of sleep _____

Exercise _____ hours   From _____ to _____

Type _____

Relaxation _____ minutes   From _____ to _____

Type_____

Meal	Time	Notes/Symptoms
Breakfast		
Morning Snack		
Lunch		
Afternoon Snack		
Dinner		
Medication		
Supplements		
Total glasses of water		
Bowel Movements		

Date: ___/___/___

Sleep   _____ hours   From _____ to _____

Quality of sleep _____

Exercise   _____ hours   From _____ to _____

Type _____

Relaxation   _____ minutes   From _____ to _____

Type_____

Meal	Time	Notes/Symptoms
Breakfast		
Morning Snack		
Lunch		
Afternoon Snack		
Dinner		
Medication		
Supplements		
Total glasses of water		
Bowel Movements		

Gratitude Affirmation

Being grateful for what I have brings more abundance into my life.

Date: ___/___/___

Sleep _____ hours   From _____ to _____

Quality of sleep _____

Exercise _____ hours   From _____ to _____

Type _____

Relaxation _____ minutes   From _____ to _____

Type_____

Meal	Time	Notes/Symptoms
Breakfast		
Morning Snack		
Lunch		
Afternoon Snack		
Dinner		
Medication		
Supplements		
Total glasses of water		
Bowel Movements		

Date: ___/___/___

Sleep _____ hours   From _____ to _____

Quality of sleep _____

Exercise _____ hours   From _____ to _____

Type _____

Relaxation _____ minutes   From _____ to _____

Type_____

Meal	Time	Notes/Symptoms
Breakfast		
Morning Snack		
Lunch		
Afternoon Snack		
Dinner		
Medication		
Supplements		
Total glasses of water		
Bowel Movements		

Personal Challenge

This evening when you get home, keep only one light on in your house at a time.

Date: ___ / ___ / ___

Sleep   _____ hours   From _____ to _____

Quality of sleep _____

Exercise   _____ hours   From _____ to _____

Type _____

Relaxation   _____ minutes   From _____ to _____

Type_____

Meal	Time	Notes/Symptoms
Breakfast		
Morning Snack		
Lunch		
Afternoon Snack		
Dinner		
Medication		
Supplements		
Total glasses of water		
Bowel Movements		

Quote

"To avoid sickness eat less; to prolong life worry less."
Chu Hui Weng

Date: ___/___/___

Sleep _____ hours From _____ to _____

Quality of sleep _____

Exercise _____ hours From _____ to _____

Type _____

Relaxation _____ minutes From _____ to _____

Type_____

Meal	Time	Notes/Symptoms
Breakfast		
Morning Snack		
Lunch		
Afternoon Snack		
Dinner		
Medication		
Supplements		
Total glasses of water		
Bowel Movements		

Gratitude Affirmation

I am eternally grateful for my mind which can solve problems.

Date: ___/___/___

Sleep   _____ hours   From _____ to _____

                         Quality of sleep _____

Exercise   _____ hours   From _____ to _____

                Type _____

Relaxation   _____ minutes   From _____ to _____

                Type_____

Meal	Time	Notes/Symptoms
Breakfast		
Morning Snack		
Lunch		
Afternoon Snack		
Dinner		
Medication		
Supplements		
Total glasses of water		
Bowel Movements		

Health Tip
Avoid carbonated drinks since carbonation is a gut irritant. Smoothies are also questionable since they have air pumped into them during the making.

Date: ___/___/___

Sleep   _____ hours   From _____ to _____

Quality of sleep _____

Exercise   _____ hours   From _____ to _____

Type _____

Relaxation   _____ minutes   From _____ to _____

Type_____

Meal	Time	Notes/Symptoms
Breakfast		
Morning Snack		
Lunch		
Afternoon Snack		
Dinner		
Medication		
Supplements		
Total glasses of water		
Bowel Movements		

Personal Challenge

Do something your future self will thank you for, like starting a savings plan.

Date: ___/___/___

Sleep   _____ hours   From _____ to _____

Quality of sleep _____

Exercise   _____ hours   From _____ to _____

Type _____

Relaxation   _____ minutes   From _____ to _____

Type _____

Meal	Time	Notes/Symptoms
Breakfast		
Morning Snack		
Lunch		
Afternoon Snack		
Dinner		
Medication		
Supplements		
Total glasses of water		
Bowel Movements		

Date: ___/___/___

Sleep _____ hours From _____ to _____

Quality of sleep _____

Exercise _____ hours From _____ to _____

Type _____

Relaxation _____ minutes From _____ to _____

Type _____

Meal	Time	Notes/Symptoms
Breakfast		
Morning Snack		
Lunch		
Afternoon Snack		
Dinner		
Medication		
Supplements		
Total glasses of water		
Bowel Movements		

Date: ___/___/___

Sleep   _____ hours   From _____ to _____

         Quality of sleep _____

Exercise   _____ hours   From _____ to _____

         Type _____

Relaxation   _____ minutes   From _____ to _____

         Type_____

Meal	Time	Notes/Symptoms
Breakfast		
Morning Snack		
Lunch		
Afternoon Snack		
Dinner		
Medication		
Supplements		
Total glasses of water		
Bowel Movements		

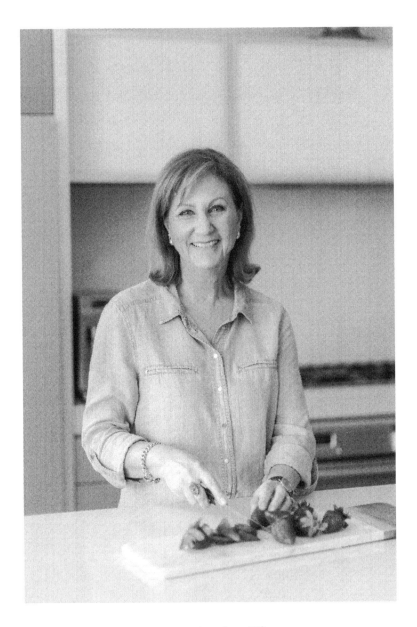

www.strandsofmylife.com
www.facebook.com/Lowfodmap

Suzanne Perazzini is also the author of two low Fodmap cookbooks, Low Fodmap Menus and Low Fodmap Snacks. She is also the creator of the successful Inspired Life Low Fodmap Coaching Program which has helped hundreds of people eliminate their IBS symptoms.

She lives in New Zealand in a house overlooking the Pacific Ocean with her husband and son. Since discovering the low FODMAP diet, her irritable bowel syndrome issues, which she has suffered from all her life, have all but disappeared.

Her blog, *Strands of my life,* focuses on the low FODMAP diet and features videos, recipes and articles on irritable bowel syndrome. Her mission in life is to help those who suffer from irritable bowel syndrome to implement the low Fodmap diet.

If you would like a complimentary, obligation-free phone call from Suzanne to discuss your issues and her coaching program, fill in the application form on this page *strandsofmylife.com/inspiredlife* and she will call you.

If you have enjoyed this book, please leave a review on Amazon.

Made in the USA
San Bernardino, CA
01 August 2017